Stretching For The Inflexible - Beginner Stretching

SADANAND PUJARI

Published by SADANAND PUJARI, 2024.

Table of Contents

Copyright

Copyright © 2024 by **SADANAND PUJARI**

Stretching For The Inflexible - Beginner Stretching

Discover The Hidden Secrets Of How To Stretch The Right Way!

First Edition: Jun 2024

Book Design by **SADANAND PUJARI**

About

Flexibility is a fundamental physical characteristic of a person. Flexibility is one of those qualities that the human body loses in the first place, and usually we do not even notice how quickly we lose the range of motion. In addition, the muscle pain that people experience, especially those who do not regularly engage in physical activity, is most often caused by the imbalance that gradually arises in the muscles.

Often this imbalance can be corrected with a properly selected stretching program, exercises that can be performed only for a few minutes a day, and not only at home, but almost anywhere.

To become a full-fledged guide in the development of flexibility.

Whatever your purpose, we hope that the suggested information will help you to improve your fitness and health.

Intro and Key Concepts

Hi everybody. It's a beginners program in stretching but even more so from people that are very inflexible like myself when I was a kid when I was 15 to 25 I was a black belt and I could stick my foot behind my head and I could do full splits inside splits and all kinds of impressive maneuvers. But between twenty five and now I'm fifty five in the last 30 years I've done nothing but desk jobs basically being a director or a therapist or a trainer it's mostly sitting behind a desk and here's what you have to do to ruin your stretch and to become totally constricted with you stretch before or not you absolutely nothing.

That's all you have to do. It's called atrophy which is where things simply degenerate over time and constriction where things tighten over time. Now I did the absolute worst thing a human being can ever do. I sat at a desk. Let me demonstrate with a chair here. Why that's such an awful basic chair here, no trick photography. You sit in a chair. Here's what happens to damage your body. We said all you could do is nothing and wait for the constriction. Now if you want to get maximum constriction make sure you don't extend any of your body parts. OK. When they're extended they're long gated and they would have a hard time constricting.

Why? Because they're extended now. How many of you sit at your desk like this? For those of you who still have a job. I'm assuming it's nobody. OK. If you do it like that your job saves the photographs. I'll get a great laugh out of it. I'll show all my friends. But if you're doing a typical desk job you've constricted your legs. So now these are gonna tighten up and you can almost see like they're seizing and place look as I try to stretch my leg. I can't get my legs straight out. That's terrible. OK your arms will do the same thing. They start getting stiff and the shoulders of the neck because you're holding it bad. Your arms are constricted; they're at an angle.

They're not out like this. They start getting tight in the biceps and across the shoulders and up through the neck especially as stress starts becoming a factor as well too. Maybe you're slouching in your chair a little bit. Now your back is curved the wrong way and starts to tighten into place so bad posture, bent knees, bent arms is probably the least of it but just hold this position for 10-20 -30 years like I did. And you will seize up totally. That's all you have to do. It's not about old age, it's not about injuries. I thought I might have some medical problem or maybe in the martial arts I tore something you know or you know maybe I had some kind of degenerative joint disease or something. No, I just had moved very little.

So I exercised and I worked out a little bit but that had absolutely nothing to do with stress. So I looked like I was in decent shape but I was totally inflexible. So now we're gonna teach you how to break out of that. So here's the first concept that I want to give you in keeping with the constriction. I'll go ahead and I'll flash up on the screen. Maybe I'll put it up on the screen over here so you can see it. This is fashion. Fashion is tissue, the spider-like web-like tissue that forms over all the muscles. If I say cut open your leg right here and flip it back. You think you see oh nice red meat like you'd see on a steak. No you wouldn't. You'd see all that fashion tissue on top. It surrounds every muscle. It's a fibrous material that holds things together.

If you look at your garden hose reel closely you think it's just this long green tube. Know what you're going to find if you look at it. There's this hex pattern like a checkerboard. It's got different fibers going through it to reinforce it. Otherwise the pressure from the water would make it bulge and eventually rupture. So to double or triple the strength of that hose they make a net around it. So you've got this net around the outside of the tubing. That's the same thing, the same kind of netting the fashion that you have around your muscles to hold them in place. It's part of what helps them to work.

But if you don't periodically stretch, which breaks up that fashion, that fashion will sit there, it'll thicken and it'll start to harden. You will start to lose its elasticity and then we start to lose our elasticity. So a couple of things that you need to do. I'll do a bonus chapter at the end to kind of show you how to break up the fashion. You can literally massage it, grind it, use rollers, and use different techniques to break up that fashion. That's one way to do it. And the second way is simply stretching. You can almost see as you're stretching. You can feel the muscles pulling and you could almost feel the fashion going click click click click click.

It's starting to break up. Why cause you pulled it beyond its ability to stretch and it starts to break up. So those are the two ways of literally grinding it. OK beating it down and stretching it out. So once you start to break that up you start to get more flexibility. So the first thing that you are going to notice is not a great stretch at first but you're going to notice that soreness starts to go away. I'm going to show you a great shoulder stretch that I do and my shoulder pain used to keep me up and waking up three times during the night and having to come out and use a massage roller.

It was an automated one that was electronic and had kind of the shot to massage with the balls and I would wrap that around my neck and push it in as hard as I could. It would just grind into those muscles. What was it doing releasing the tension in the muscles and breaking up the fashion? And that was the only thing that stopped the pain. But after just three days of doing this very simple stretching exercise with my shoulders gone and never ever returned even though I don't do that stretch that much anymore I might do that stretch once a week or once a month doesn't matter because I broke up all that fashion tissue and I trained my body not to tense that way anymore. By what.

Gently stretching it every once in a while. So I'm going to break down these chapters. So we're doing just one, two , maybe three techniques, maybe a fourth technique, so it's nice we'll just do one. I want to explain it well. I don't want it to be like one of these aerobics exercise chapters where they're jumping around and hey they show you something three or four times and by about the fourth time you've got it on the fifth time they go into the next exercise. You may not have even got it yet. I want this slow and simple and broken down so you can see it perform it with me or stop the tape. Take some time to do it yourself. But I'm not going to be jumping on to the next thing. This is not an exercise chapter. This is a stretching chapter.

I want you to get the technique. I don't want you to get a workout. I'm here basically dressed in a polo shirt and that's about what you need as long as you can move around and get some baggy pants and something you can move around your upper body. That's fine. You don't need a special workout outfit. We're not going to stretch that hard. We're not getting exercise clothes because we're not going to break a sweat. Very simple, very delicate. Stretch it. And I've got two chairs you can see I'm on either side of me. They're my favorite tool. Why? Because anytime I need an assist something's a little too much. I'm stretching over to the side.

Oh even that's too much weight. You can do a couple of things if you're doing a stretch like this. You can take your arm down and just go like this because now you're not putting this extra weight up above you could put your hand on your hip to help ease things down or you could use the chair. So there's different stages. I want you to do gentle stretching. Hold the stretching. This is not something that builds up muscle. This is the build up stretch. And I don't want you to overdo it. So typical disclaimer OK I'm not a licensed physical therapist I'm not a doctor at least not that kind.

Right. So check in with your doctor. This is not medical advice. This is for educational purposes. If anything hurts, stop checking with your doctor first and the six other disclaimers I haven't thought of. OK I'll put them at the beginning of the chapter. But go gentle, go easy , go slow now. Last thing I want to tell you before I end this beginning chapter is go slow. The tortoise wins the race. If you're holding a stretch and you're doing it about say maybe 60 percent of what you can do that will make sure you're not sore the next day. If you try to do 70-80 90 percent of what you could do you may get a little more stretch and be very proud of yourself today. But then you're going to hurt your leg. And if you're sore the next day and the next day and the next day the next day that's for days that you can't stretch it's four days you're behind you may have even injured the muscle. OK so maybe temporary some might be permanent.

Who knows how bad you did it and you've lost your progress, you've lost your momentum. It's going to start to seize up again so slow and steady. This is a game of inches in millimeters. Little tiny bit every single day. Slow progress even some plateaus once in a while. The first thing you do is get rid of stiffness and we want to get a little bit of a stretch and then we're going to progress in our stretch. Then you could do the more advanced stretches in some other exercise chapter with the girl in the pretty leotard sticking her foot behind her head. If you want to go that far, that's great. But this is for people like me so elderly people and flexible people, maybe even people with injuries, really check with your doctor and your physical therapist if you have injuries. Remember this is just an educational chapter just for questions. This is not medical advice in any way shape or form but go ahead and join us and I'll see you in the very next chapter.

Understanding Static Stretching

Now the first thing you want to do is rule number one don't stretch COLD MUSCLES COLD MUSCLES tear warm muscles stretch when I just say COLD MUSCLES tear war muscles stretch. So how can you warm up the muscles. Most relaxing way that I like to do it is I like to go for a nice walk. You want to get a little bit warmer so that you can jog a little bit. I used to do some jumping jacks and I wanted to do something that was lower impact while still doing the jumping jacks. I did the elliptical machine. Very low impact. Love the elliptical machine but boy it really works the legs. I've also got a little recumbent bike so I can do that as well. That's even gentler and easier than the elliptical machine.

But Of course I can always set the tension. You can just do leg raises. I'll just do the leg races that would warm it up or even lunge a little bit side to side. Anything that warms up the muscles you're going to be doing the upper body stretches and we do a few of those then I would just lift some gentle hand weights or grab a half gallon of milk or something or some soup cans whatever is a good weight for you and just move those to get the arms going. Now once you've warmed up the upper and the lower body you remember whenever you warm up one part you pretty much warm up the other one because if I were doing squats with a weight Yeah I'm working the heck out of my legs but my whole body is hot.

Why is my four heads sweating because it goes through the entire body. How best to do a little bit of exercise that does work the upper body does work the lower body but any exercise even like I said go for a walk. It's going to have some effect across the body. So those are your basic warm up exercises. You do any kind of warm up exercises that you like. Long as it does a little bit of the upper body and more so on the lower body because this is where you are going to be doing probably 20 percent of your stretching. And this is where you are going to be doing maybe 80 percent of your stretching. Most people probably have flexibility from the waist down not from the waist up. So warm body stretches cold body tethers. Now we also want to work the joints to warm up the insides of the joints. How do we do that?

Just think about what joints you're going to be using and how they move. So a lot of times they'll start with neck rolls or back and forth with the neck side to side with the neck. Just move it any way you can think of. That'll warm up the neck and start to stretch that out. That's actually a key area a lot of people get a stiff neck just doing that. We'll give you a gentle stretch because it's hard to move it without stretching it a little bit because my neck is so stiff right now. I was working out the other day. It's really stiff. Sometimes you just take a finger or two fingers and just move it over a little bit. Roll the shoulders a little bit so the neck is the first joint, shoulders are the second joint. How can you move your shoulders? Shoulders basically move up and they move down.

So this is a good warmup for it right. They also move up and down in this direction to them in that direction and they go round around do it in this direction turn sideways and do it either or that's about all there is to a shoulder warmup. Now the next thing is the spine in the hips. You turn to one side you turn to the other you turn to one side you turn to the other you can lean back a little bit you can lean forward a little bit you can kick it out to one side a little bit you can kick it out to the other side a little bit you can roll it that's about it you just gently warming it up you can also hold on to something like the chair use the chairs quite a bit and just rotate the leg inside the hip great way to do it grab another chair.

That's why I always like to practice for balance. Go one finger with the chair when you get better and your balance gets better. Like this for a lot of people have balance issues that can help a lot to improve their balance. Pretty soon they don't need your cane anymore. OK now the knees are the next joint. Think of it this way. How do I move the knee? I move it like this. OK. And it'll go a little bit. Side side so I basically just go like this a few times and I kick it out kick it out straight from the side a little bit. That's it. Then I'll go a little bit to one side and a little bit to the other. Then I find your strength. And then what I do is I take my knees and I just roll in this direction. Pretty simple, pretty basic and I'm kind of going up and down a little bit. That's it. Nothing too exciting.

Sometimes I'd bend the man and bend them out. That's about it. Now you've warmed up the joints. Now your body's ready to do the first stretches so let's do some real simple stretches just to get the body in the stretching move. So the first thing I do is I usually go off to one side. Then I go off to the other then to the other then to the other almost like I'm just warming up the hips again but I'm trying to get a little bit of straps I may grab onto something. And again just very gentle pressure, maybe like two fingers just to get a light stretch. You can use the chair again if you need to use that to kind of pull yourself around a little bit. Just two fingers and that's it. It's all a stretch you want then I want to stretch it side to side because that's where most people get stiff.

Sup use the chair if you need to. So one way to do it is just over like this. But then you're putting all of this weight and all your body weight and nothing supporting it's really going to pull here. If you want less weight put one hand on the hit that'll support it and you can go over like this if you want less weight than that take the hand away if you want less weight than that used to chair. See I can always adjust these to your fitness level. Then just do the other side and again once you feel a light stretch Hold it. This is known as static stretching. Don't bounce. There's a lot of controversy. Some people can bounce lightly if they do it very slowly and rhythmically if they're very well stretched and they agree they can.

I wouldn't. Why? Because bouncing could hurt you. STATIC STRETCH readers come over and you hold it literally can't. Never seen any scientific research where that hurt you. So the longer you hold any one of these stretches the better off you're going to be. So that's your next strategy. Think of it this way. I'm already here. I already got the clothes on and you got the chair out. I'm ready to exercise. I CAN HOLD THIS STRETCH FOR FIVE SECONDS. ONE TWO THREE FOUR FIVE. Or I can go over and I can hold it for 15 seconds. Only it takes me 10 seconds longer. It might extend say my 15 minutes stretching routine into 20 minutes to double my stretching time but I'll also double my results.

Let me be a little bit more than double. So why are you there , especially if you're inflexible? Hold it for longer. This gives the muscles time to relax to release and what you're doing with stretching is your muscles could stretch; they could release if they wanted to weigh more than they do. Most people don't realize if the fascist properly broke up you could drop right now into a split. No problem. Why? Because a full split is a hundred percent of your range of motion. Your muscles actually have a hundred and twenty to one hundred and thirty percent range of motion. So you could actually put like two Boston phone books on either side and go all the way down to this floor in the full splitter side split and that would be about one hundred and thirty percent. Why is it that I can only stretch about this far. OK. Why?

Because the muscles are not trained to do that so they tighten up. It's almost like if you were under hypnosis you could do it but your unconscious mind. Because it's not trained to believe you can do the full split it can't do it. So a lot of stretching is mental. So the longer you hold the static stretch it says hey I can stretch at least this far and I know I can because every second I'm doing and I'm at hand doing it I'm doing it I'm doing it I'm doing it. And then your body believes you can do what you can do. And it says OK almost like a thermostat that you're slowly ticking up. He remembers the last setting and the next day goes up another degree another degree another degree. So you do this in literally fractions of an inch. Mm. A little bit more each day.

That's how you're going to get all the way down a little bit at a time each day and hold it to lock in those gains. So the longer you do it the more you lock in the gains. So a lot of people want to do it for long periods of time. They'll pick out maybe the 20 or so stretches that I'll show you. They'll pick five or six for their worst problem areas or the areas they just want to have a nice gain in and what they'll do is they'll do a simple stretch you know maybe like a hamstring stretch like this but they'll do it while they're sitting on the caps so their butts on the couch they're sitting like this. They get into a position where they can feel some tension there. That's about 60 percent or 70 percent of what they can do for a stretch and they hold it there. How long.

Minute two minutes three minutes four minutes. I'll be leaving within five minutes but usually between 30 seconds and three minutes is considered a long gated stretch that will really lock it in. Now it will be boring to sit going through all 20 stretches and hold it for three to five minutes each. That would be too long now to do it for 10 or 20 or 15 seconds, maybe even 30 seconds or a minute. That's not too bad. You know when you're doing say a dozen different stretches but three minutes times it doesn't. Wow you're out too. Well it's almost forty five minutes. You know you're out like 35 to 40 minutes. That's a long time. It's so boring but at night and you're sitting there and you're watching TV and you just get into the stretch and you hold it. And I'm sitting here and watching TV. It's not boring at all.

That's how you do it. That's the best way to do it. You do it the way that you like. Now let's do the next stretch. The next stretch is going to be a simple HAMSTRING STRETCH. So literally the one I just showed you put your leg out. Now interestingly enough you can lock it in place like you see here the knee is completely straight and then you want to just keep yourself along to get it. This is how bad my stretch is. That's plenty of attention for me. Isn't that funny it doesn't even look like I'm bending over here's me straight up. Here's me stretching it. That's how tight my legs are. I really need this. OK. Now I could bend over and hunch my back and make it look like I'm getting really close or do something like that.

That's what most people do. Now keep it nice and straight. Doesn't matter where you are. This is the before picture that's going to make the after picture so impressive. About 60 percent of what you can do is OK. Hold it. Now if you're in as bad a shape as I am, I should probably hold it for about 30 seconds to a minute. If you really want to get the full benefit like I said, do it while watching TV or something. Do it for three minutes and then go to the next leg. Now interestingly enough you can actually bend the leg a little bit and then go a little farther and you'll still feel it in the hamstrings. If you feel your leg underneath here you can feel the hamstrings and that's still a stretch but your legs are not locked out. It's just two different styles of stretching.

Think of it this way. One of the reasons I want to get more flexible is I thought it was embarrassing as a guy with a black belt and come food that I couldn't touch my toes and I said look look I can't touch my toes and is a joke so they said well you're doing it wrong you get a bend at the knee. So I bent at the knee and I said Oh yeah. Look, I can touch my toes. I guess it was a technique issue. Now the funny thing is that's actually a stretch. You can go ahead and bend your knees and touch your toes and then kind of just pull the knees in a little bit and try to flex them out a little bit. And that's a stretch. Just go to where you get the stretch and you can stretch it like that or you can do it here.

And I would use the chair assist because remember this isn't an exercise of putting your whole upper body weight in competing against your back muscles to see if you can tell him or not it's to put the right amount of weight out in the right amount of stretch. So for hamstring stretches like this or you're trying to even do toe touches I don't care what your level is I would pretty much use the chair unless you're at the expert level. Those are a couple different hamstring stretches. In the next chapter we'll show you some more stretches to make it even more flexible.

Stretching Secrets

Hey, welcome back everybody. In a previous chapter we were showing you how to do the hamstring stretches and we basically showed you how to do them here with the assistance of the chair. Put them out here. They can also do different levels. So what you should do is you should have something like the chair and let me grab my phone. BLOCK Now what I'm going to do is instead of going here and maybe go into here stretching this far over I'll go here but not stretch as far here. So it's two different stretches. One of the lower levels is a little higher than a little higher than a little higher. So there's two ways to stretch by leaning forward and create tension here. And by raising the legs slowly I like to do a little bit of both. They give you slightly different stretches as you raise a little bit higher.

It gets a little farther down on the hamstring OK more to the groin area. OK. And when you're here it gets more down in this area towards the knee. So two different styles. You get a little bit different stretch. Perfect blocks are great. These foam blocks are called Yoga blocks. You can use them for different stretches especially when you're really inflexible but you're trying to get flexible. This is another aid just like a chair. So say you were doing full splits but you couldn't quite get down there to where you could put your palms down enough to be off the floor. Well I can raise it by a block or I can turn it this way and raise it even more. OK.

I could put two yoga blocks here whatever I need or go back to the chair. So these are just a nice little spacer to add those levels that you need to take the pressure off of the stretch or to slowly increase your stretch. These are like a six to eight dollar item on Amazon. So I would definitely get the yoga blocks. Now the other stretch that you can do is from the side and you simply put your foot up here. You want to keep your toes pointing like I'm pointing towards you and all you want to do is just kind of go over. It's gonna work the hips, it's going to stretch across the back. You tip your head and leave your neck a little bit.

It will work here. You'll feel it in here across the inside groin. They call us the doctors and that works the inside of the leg. We just worked the hamstrings which were the backside of the leg. We're gonna work the inside of a leg very simply again if you need help yourself with the chair put in the hand over the head can help. Sometimes that's too heavy. You put the hand on the hip. Whatever adjustment you need to make. So I hope you're getting the theory more so than the stretch allows these stretches of very common stretches that you may or may not need me to show you. It's the way in which we're doing the stretches that I want you to learn some ways and send me a comment. So this was way too simple. Yes.

Matter of fact it's very hard to find complicated stretches even at the most advanced level. So you know I saw one lady wrapped herself into the shape of a tool. That was about the most advanced thing I'd ever seen. But she's a fitness expert gymnast. You know since the age of six we're probably not going to get there. OK. Now one of the things that you can do is what's called active stretching. We said this was static stretching where you stretch a little bit. You just hold it. It's static. You're not moving dynamic stretching or moving stretching is like this. I may do the same thing. I'm going to work the hamstrings except instead of putting it up on the chair here's what I do to get a swing leg. This is on the upswing and is pulling on the hamstring.

This is a dynamic stretch. This warms the muscles, the hips work the muscles that support the stretch a little bit which is good. Lot of people don't realize that all part of the reason why they can't stretch very well is for the muscle to stretch; it needs strength in the opposing muscle. So let me teach you a trick while I'm teaching you this theory. Say I'm trying to do this stretch and I want to improve my hamstring stretch underneath here. How do I do that? A static stretching be dynamic stretching sea by strengthening this. So if I worked the quads that's these top muscles here on your thigh. If I work those then these muscles underneath will relax. Why because your muscles here are pulling against these muscles. When these muscles are stronger than this one doesn't feel like it has to pull to support when these are weak.

This will pull very tight to support the leg. So a trick that you can do in stretching is actually pushing out on the chair right now pushing up pushing up pushing down the chair. If I push down about 50 percent as hard as I can push and I hold that for about 30 seconds I will not only strengthen this muscle the opposing one which will help my stretch long term I'm also fatiguing that muscle so that after the 30 seconds when I release it my legs tired and it's easier to stretch. That's a great trick. I know a guy who sold a kid on this and that's all he did.

He pushed out, pushed out, pushed down fatigue of that muscle both by working it out and then holding it down for 30 seconds to 60 seconds and really wearing out that muscle the opposing muscle and then just stretching the opposite muscle in this case the hamstring fatigue it held for 30 seconds pushed and pushed and pushed out. Relaxing breath on the outward breath and going down breathing is very important for stretching. When you breathe when your body gets energy when you breathe out it releases energy when you breathe then it takes in energy which is tension and when you breathe out it releases energy which is relaxation. So a lot of people you'll see them breathing as if stretching on the way down. I got a friend. You always see little pursed lips, so cute looks so pretty when she does it and that's what she's doing. She does the balancing thing but every time she balances you just see her lips pressed as she goes where she knows she could touch your head to the floor.

But that's what she's doing. Even at her level it's the breath and the relaxation. A lot of what's happening is you are tensing against the you fighting it because you picture tense muscles as pain and we move away from pain. So when you're in pain you tend to tighten up the muscle if you tighten up the muscle then it won't stretch and if it's not stretching and it's not hurting so your brain kind of plays a trick on you it tightens up so you won't pull forward but your goal is to pull forward the fact that it's tightening increases the pain which makes you want to stretch even less and you get a terrible stretch but by relaxing into this stretch and breathing into the stretch you get past that mental trick of your body tightening up it's tightening up to try to relieve your pain but it's actually causing the pain things by tightening you won't push forward. If I just push against you you won't push towards me. And actually that's what you're trying to do. So the trick is to relax , release and breathe. And then just hope wherever you're comfortable that's it. OK. That's your chapter for this chapter and I'll see you in the very next one. Take care.

The Secret Of Nerve Flossing (Part 1)

Now I'm going to show you yet another type of stretching. And again these aren't necessarily unique stretches although the next couple will be. These are called neural or Nerve Flossing. I think Nerve Flossing is more accurate. So what you're doing is we talked about a static stretch. We've talked about a dynamic moving stretch and now we're looking at Nerve Flossing which means kind of moving the tendon moving the nerves as opposed to pulling on them. So it's a different kind of dynamic stretch and what it does is it affects the nerves more so than the muscle tissue in the tendon because the nerves are part of the equation as well. So think of it as just a different style of dynamic stretching.

And this will help you get gains that you otherwise wouldn't get almost all the stretch as you see when you're taking a stretching chapter about static stretching static stretching and the occasional dynamic one which almost happens by mistake. So we've shown you the static and how to do it properly. We've shown you the dynamic how to do it properly. Now I can teach you a unique system called Nerve Flossing which is a moving stretch. It's OK. So fortunately they do. ALL WE'RE GONNA DO IS WE'RE GONNA GET DOWN ON THE FLOOR AND WE'RE GONNA GET OUR KNEES up to about a 90 degree angle so straight here straight here and we're going to point our toes.

We'll do two legs and then all we're going to do is just rotate the legs a little bit and you can feel it gliding when you grab your hamstrings. That's why it's called Nerve Flossing. You can feel the hamstrings moving at the same time they're pulling almost all the time at least on the second half from here to here. I'm getting a nice pull but they're moving and sliding up and down. That's the flossing just like you would do back and forth in your teeth simply go like this you want to get a little support you can hold it and that's it. That's one style under flossing. Now reset the camera and I'll show you a second way to do it.

The Secret Of Nerve Flossing (Part 2)

OK. Welcome back everybody. Now I want to show you what must be the simplest form of Nerve Flossing ever created. It's a great stretch. I must show it to you right now. Simply sit up straight and back up against the back of the chair which you lay out as straight as you can. You can see I can't get my way up here so I'm going to go at an angle but I'm able to lock out my leg. I couldn't do it there. I just simply moved a little further in my chair. OK. I can hit it right about there. That's good. Now all I'm going to do is point my toe out and put my toe in as I'm pulling in. This would be the breathing part. And if he felt back here once again you could feel the tension sliding so you can feel this down in your calf.

You could feel it all the way up the back of the leg into the hamstring and that's all you do see how nice and gentle and easy that is nice dynamic Nerve Flossing stretch moving the tendons moving the nerves moving the muscle all at once you want you can hold it for a couple of seconds that to you on it breathing during a tense phase. Then read that for you then read that that's it. So splint is so simple and just change BE NICE GENTLE STRETCH. Anybody can do it. Perfect so that's your very next strategy. And I'll see you in the next chapter.

The Secret Of Nerve Flossing (Part 3)

Hey everybody. I love showing people how to do the Nerve Flossing. So here's another nerve flossing technique for you. Now everybody knows this typical hamstring stretch where you try to go down and touch your toes. We're going to do something similar but we're going to add Nerve Flossing. We want the muscle, the tendons, the tissue and the nerves to flow back and forth. OK. So what we're gonna do is we're gonna bend at the knee a little bit. Just put our heel into the ground, toes up and then we're gonna go but out just up just out and we're just going to go up and down a little bit with our toe point reading on the downward stroke and as you do this rocking motion very gentle very smooth again don't pull too tight.

What you're doing is if you could see inside on the other side you are just sliding everything back and forth in this area. So you're getting in the back of the calf you're getting in the hamstring area and it's just sliding gently back and forth as you drop down as you rocket it's sliding back and forth. That's why it's called Nerve Flossing. Do that a few times. That'll get you a nice stretch all the way through here and I'll tell you I feel a little bit my quad. You feel a little bit in your knee again if you need to. You can hold yourself with a chair but that's another style and Nerve Flossing again. Feel your body sense your body you'll know if you're in the right position you're doing it right because it'll feel right you'll feel that nice gentle glide that NICE GENTLE STRETCH. Don't pull too much. Again about 60 percent of what you can handle slow increments every day and you'll do fantastic. I'll see you in the next chapter.

Magic Of The Bear-Hug Stretch

Hey, welcome back everybody. Now I want to teach you one of my favorite stretches and the introductory chapter. I've talked a little bit about how I had shoulder pain and oh it would wake me up in the middle of the night. It was too much being hunched over a computer all day and just doing nothing for 30 years. Like we've talked about it was just a lot of stress at work too tight and tight and tight and and you're holding it in that position. Everything's kind of bunched up and held there under stress. Not good. So the shoulder pain got really bad until I learned a very simple stretch I call it the bear hug stretch all you do is you grab yourself like this and I want you to just go around in a circle you lean to one side and then you just start going in a circle very slowly like this and you will feel the stretch all the way across your back literally from the tip of your scapula. Is this wing bone back here all the way down to your rear end now your table and that will loosen all that up.

And this is great because you're getting the entire back. You're breaking up all that fascist tissue and you get a nice stretch across your back. If you have lower back pain and shoulder pain this is a great one. So lean to one side. Roll it around. I feel so good. I usually get a nice stretch on either end and just shake it out a little bit. Feels great. Let me show you the same thing. Give yourself a big hug. Start at one side. Just what your body can handle. I want you sensing your back. What's the right amount of attention for you if this is too heavy for you again. Just kind of keep you could almost go like this and support yourself with your arms. Doesn't work quite as well but it takes the weight off.

OK. Or you can lean back a little bit more and then go into it. And that would take some of the weight off as well. Bad posture but that's OK I feel so good.

Whoo. Nice. You can do it. Kind of one arm at a time if you want to just go across. You could just pull it here a little bit. You go across and pull it here a little bit but you don't get that nice wave across the shoulders. I love this because I just get a wave of stretch heels just like a wave going across my back and then I go the other way and it's another wave. All those tents, all those tendons and all that fashion, all that musculature all the way down the back relaxing releasing feels fantastic. That stretch alone should be worth what you paid for the Book. Like I said it got rid of the muscular tension in my shoulders. It helped to alleviate the frozen shoulder issue that I had and it stopped me from waking up at night. It relieved a lot of pain for me. Relieve a lot of pain for you that you did for today and I'll see you in the very next chapter.

Shoulder and Trapezius Stretch

Hey everybody. Now we're gonna show you how to stretch out the shoulders again. How we're doing it is as important if not more important than the technique. You could jump onto YouTube and find all kinds of stretching chapters but you're not going to find the science and techniques that you're finding here. So one of the first things we want to do is think about how to stretch your shoulders. I used to do a funny thing where I would show people hand techniques. It was how to grapple with people. And I call the technique doesn't go like that. So if you want to figure out how to grapple something you start at the far end of the finger.

And what I would do is I'd say if you want to control somebody just make their fingers go the way they don't go. How can you control somebody then their thumb back like this because it doesn't go like this. See how they immediately have to move their entire body then bend their fingers back like this. Then take all their fingers and bend it back like this. Then take the thumb and take it and hyperextend it the other way. Don't go like that. Then start working your way up the risk doesn't go like that doesn't go like that and you can start manipulating people. So what you think about in the shoulder is which way does it move and which way do I get a stretch. And then you'll be able to come up with your own stretches. So think of it this way.

One of the things that we said the shoulder does is it goes up and down like this. So one of the things that I want you to do is take a wall and literally just crawl your fingers up the wall to where you get a good stretch. When you get a good stretch try to carve up a smidge more and maybe lean into it and lean away from it a little bit lean into it and lean away from it a little bit go up a little bit farther. Feel the stretch maybe get a little more stretch by dropping now while you're there and leaning towards the wall that actually gives the nicest stretch. Then once you get a little bit stretched out see things go up a little bit further. Again don't do more than 60 percent of what you figure you can do better to hold it for longer periods of time than to stretch it more.

Remember that it is better to hold it longer than to stretch it farther. I'd rather you went 60 percent of the way you could go and held it for a minute then you went Sixty five percent as far as you can go and held it for 10 seconds or even held it for a minute but then hurt yourself and put yourself back several days don't do that. So this is the first one which is going to give you this range in motion obviously. Yep. Now the other way it goes is just across so you can pull your arm here or you can put your arm across something and then just turn into it gently turn into it just hold it lock put your hand there if you need to and just move into it very gently again you can hold it or you can do a dynamic where I'm just very gently moving back and forth don't bounce like one of these don't bounce like that but a smooth roll that you can do nice smooth roll that you can do but I tend to just stretch it hold it wait hold it release shake it out move it around do it a little bit more then go the next stretch.

Now as you're doing this one you've actually got different angles of stretch. This is where it becomes unique. So you do it here then you do it here then you do it here then you do it here and you do it here. Same exact motion, different levels it's going down through. And then I'm going to go below where I started and turn it in as you go really low you have to get a little closer to the wall right that works at every possible angle within this range. So now we did it this way and now we did it across the body at all the different angles that starts activating different stretches of different muscles. You'll feel it. People go like this and they say oh I stretched it across here and I'm done now. I usually go like one two three four five So middle two above two below.

That gives me five different stretches. That's usually plenty but I've seen people that evolve you know an inch at a time. They really like to refine it and get a hell of a stretch if you do it like that. OK. Now next stretch your arm goes up and it goes over so what you can do is just simply grab your elbow and give it a light stretch. Some people will use a resistance band where they'll grab on to the resistance band and then they'll pull it back here. You can do that. That's a little bit more advanced. OK. Normally even just sometimes the weight of your arm is enough like that or just again a couple of fingers very gently. And again you can even move it out and in a slightly different stretch depending upon how you're doing it way out here. Weigh in here a little bit differently. OK. Now that's pushing it about as far this way as it goes. How about if we go as far this way as it goes. Well the easiest way to do it is to start with something that has levels.

I like this because it has levels but you could use a short chair you know or a coffee table you know or say your dining room table. Then you could use maybe the back of a chair then you could use the top of your couch you know whatever you have. You'll get creative, you'll find things. I just use my entertainment center. So

I will start with this one. And if I want to get a stretch all I do is I go down a little bit to get the stretch when I get stretched out. If I go to the next level then I do go down a little bit more. OK here's another legitimate cheat. Remember our old friend the yoga block says I've only got one level. Great. Put that there. Put the yoga block there. Now I have gained a little more height. I can flip the yoga block up.

Now I'm still a little taller. How did one level become three? It's like the loaves and fishes. I got my yoga block. So the yoga block is a great strategy to give you small increments literally of about two to four inches at a time. So this is about four inches here. This is about six inches here and that's why I say about two to four inches perfect. Matter of fact if you want to think about it I think it's eight inches across so you could go like four six and then eight. It's a little less dirty when you do it that way. OK. Now one of the things that I like to do to warm up the shoulders is do something that's called dynamic tension. This is the old classic Charles Atlas. The guy comes and kicks sand in your face at the beach. OK.

What he would do is he would take one muscle against the other and just strain it so you could do one muscle against the other. You can really feel that in the shoulders. I'm pulling with one against the other. I could also push with one against the other. This is a nice warm up. Great to warm the muscles before you stretch. Remember warm muscle stretch cold muscles tear you can also do this with nothing. I can push this way and I can push this way. This is muscle against muscle within the arm. I'm just kind of imagining a weight there but I'm actually tensing one muscle against the other. So you can really see it in the triceps there when I do it. The triceps activate the goal. If you're doing a curl. Same thing now you're warming up the arm when muscles against the other you're overhead do it like you're lifting a weight over your head.

Bull activates all the shoulders and warms them up. OK. So warm up, stretch and relax and breathe. Just stretch. Now you also want to go across the body. We talked about doing it like this. You can also use a tool for that. I usually just put my hand on the wall and I twist it this way and I put my hand against the wall and I twist it this way and I'll tell you. That's about every stretch you ever need to work all the shoulders. We taught you the bear hug stretch to get from the shoulders on down. So now you've done the entire area, the shoulder all the way around the other muscle that you need to get in here. You get that mostly with the bare stretch but you can also do that just by pulling down here and pulling down here.

You also feel that right across here this one is the trash piece that's called. It's just this muscle here. This whole shoulder muscle up here is the upper shoulder muscle as opposed to the lower shoulder muscle. Just a good massage is the best way to loosen that up. There's no real way to really stretch that muscle that muscle is most likely to release if you exercise it and fatigue is the way to do that is all those muscles do is they move your shoulders up and down so you know what the exercise for that is move your shoulders up move your shoulders down move your shoulders up move your shoulders down a lot of times if you do it with a sigh. Bring them up tight. 10 releases. Bring them up quickly. Bring them up quick drop in an exhale like you're saying.

That's the best way to release the trip. Easiest muscles that you tip for today and I'll see you in the next chapter.

Groin Stretch - Inner Thigh

Hey, welcome back everybody. Now I want to show you some SIDE STRETCH ones. This would kind of be a lead up to doing side splits but I don't think we'll even get that far. Not that kind of chapter but I do want you to be able to work the inner groin muscles a little bit because that's about the only one that we've only done a little bit of work on. So to strengthen the legs a little bit and to get a stretch. Hope you can see this with it with the chair in the way. I basically put my hands on the chair and all they do and that's why I got socks on a slippery floor. It's just letting that leg go out until it locks and I'm bending this knee and just getting a little bit of stretch right in here in the groin area. Very light, very gentle.

Just what it can handle and then you hold it for a few seconds you let it back in. If you want to do a flossing exercise you can do a smooth in and out just like you're just rubbing the floor with your foot. Even the floor a little massage with your foot nice that's it. Then you switch sides. And you can hold it when you've got more time. I don't want to you know demonstrate a three minute Holder 30 second home hold foot and that's as much or as little as you can do. That'll give you good strength in the quads which we said will help you work the opposite side. It's going to give you a good stretch on the doctors. So the perfect stretch is very well supported. Make sure you don't slip. Make sure you got a good sturdy chair. That's all you need to do this stretch. Take care.

Benefits Of Yoga Stretching

Hey everybody, welcome back. Now I'm going to show you a little bit of yoga. Just the simplest of yoga. Now what is yoga? Yoga is just simply the stretching of the muscles. It's what they call studio yoga. There's two kinds of yoga. Yoga is where you go to a higher mental level. That's one form of yoga. Then there's studio yoga which is all about the stretching and the positions versus the spiritual aspect. So we're going to be looking at the stretching and the positions, not the spiritual aspect that means a totally different chapter. So I want to show you that it's not this weird ancient mystical art. It's simply movement and stretching and that's all we're gonna do we're gonna do the simplest yoga stretches known to man and anybody can do all I can do you can do.

So first of all we're going to simply do the CAT STRETCH SO YOU GET IN THIS POSITION HERE AND THEN you arch your back up then bring your head forward and arched it out stretching especially the lower back and then that out there. Now if you want in any position you can just kind of work it around a little bit. Move your hips, move your shoulders, loosen stuff up. I like to extend it out and then wiggle it because it gives me a good stretch on my shoulders and on my back. You can even go back and forth like this. This is actually called child pose. They just go down here and they stretch across the back. So that's the second pose. Feels really good.

And that's all you do. Nice and gentle work shifts like this a little bit. You'll get a little bit more stretch. This is just a rolling technique perfect back here. Now they've got a position where you go sweeping through and they do a downward dog. All I do is I get my butt down to the mat and I'm just going to lie down like I'm taking a nap for the day. I'm going to put my hands by my side and I'm going to see how much. Usually right around between when you're facing your shoulder is I'm just going to push and see if I get a little curve on my back just to flex the back a little bit a little stretch in the back. You can even put your elbows down.

This is what I do when I want to hold it. Just getting a stretch in the back and then I do the rolling technique that loosens up stuff in the back and in the hips. You move your shoulders and he loosens things up in the shoulders. All I'm doing. Whatever level you can get to. You can't go that high. Then you go here. I mean you can do it a lot of different ways and just do it here. I mean you can set any level you want. You could use the yoga blocks. I'm. My back is very stiff. I had several back injuries. This is about what I can do so I imagine if you're like 50 like me and even 60 or 70 or 80 if you had no back injury you could probably do this. That's it. That's one stretch. This is two stretches that's the CAT STRETCH.

Child's Pose nice pull on the back from here. Lot of people just go in different directions. Sometimes a nice hand movement is good. Just like you walking around stretch here. STRETCH HERE. PUT YOUR HAND HERE IN A HAND HERE. TURN A LITTLE BIT TO THIS WAY. HERE and HERE and HERE. Wherever you can get. You can't grab the mat whatever you got to do wherever you can grab it just a gentle stretch in this way. STRETCH TO THIS SIDE STRETCH

TO THIS SIDE STRETCH TO THIS SIDE STRETCH TO THIS SIDE GET DOWN AND GO GRAB YOU DO THAT YOU'LL HAVE WONDERFUL flexibility all around the middle area which is the spine that's the area that tends to get the most tight even that's a good stretch is moving it around you like figure eights with your shoulders anything you can do that you feel loosens it up you're doing it right. Just move it in different ways, feel where it's tight for you, sense your body, listen to your body, go slow , and take your time.

Make sure you warm up first all the things that we've been teaching you but see all those poses are so simple they're not complicated but they do a huge amount of what the remaining poses do especially for what you need if you're not going to be a yoga instructor you're not a professional athlete you're not going to be Superman jumping over tall buildings you don't need this for any particular reason except you want better health and you want to be able to move well as a normal human being and not be in pain not have tension not having the infirmities of old age you just want to be fluid and healthy and alive and this is plenty what I've shown you everything above that is for some kind of specific task athletic performance or maybe a job requirement you do a lot of heavy lifting and you need know more stretching and strength around your back or in your legs or something like that but otherwise a lot of exercises that they show you out on the web on the Internet in the gyms and things like this they actually have nothing to do with what a human being is going to do during the Book of their day they serve no other function than building up muscle for I don't know for vanity for parents and just something to do away you're at the gym. That's your tip for today. That's your new strategy your new technique that's going to help create a new you. Thanks so much.

Tools To Release Fascia & Tension

Hi everybody. I know you may have just seen me seconds ago but for me it's been about an hour and a half. Why? I've been trying to find a few simple tools and I want to share them with you today. But my wife hit him. Now if you ever come up with a chapter of how to get a wife to stop hiding things in the house from their husband I'll buy your trading Book. Now the first thing is a roller bar. There's actually a technique called I believe it's called Gow shore. I always mispronounce it but it's basically breaking up that fashion tissue by using tools to dig in and they really dig it. It's called scraping. Why? Because they take the tools and they scrape against the skin and the muscles and it turns beet red.

You will bruise there's some blood vessels that may get broken or teeth. I mean they're really grinding in to break that fashion to break it up around the muscle. For some people that have really set in fashion tissue in their muscles they just need to really get in there and grind it. Now there's some massage therapists that'll do fashion releases and that's what they're doing. If you've ever had a deep tissue massage just multiply that by five. And that's what it takes to break up that fashion. And they'll do it by stretching, pulling , tearing at it, rolling it back and forth between their fingers basically any way they can really dig in there and break it apart. And the other way to do it very gently and won't be as invasive and won't be as intense and it won't be as thorough but you can do it through something called rolling now rolling can be done a couple different ways.

I've got a couple of different tools here for you. I've got a classic foam roller and what people will do with this is they'll simply put their weight against it like lie on the floor and then they roll back and forth on the floor and let it hit the different areas. You do the front. You do the back, you do the side. You can do your shoulders, you can do your arms, you can do inside, you can do outside. You can do a cross you know the middle of your back. You can roll it but rolling is simply putting pressure on your body. Any body part against the roller and then going back and forth and that just crushes the fashion and helps to break it up. Some people even roll a little bit this way as opposed to just like this.

So when they have their leg on it they roll their leg across it a little bit. And a lot of times what people will do is they'll really work on or even hold and grind it too and apply extra pressure to certain areas that are really tight to create a release. So some people will do this before stretching or working out. Some people will do it after stretching or working out. So it helps for stretching, helps for fashion release and it also helps to release some tense blocked areas. That's kind of an old massage technique. You can massage something by manipulating it and moving it. You can massage something by stretching it as technique number two and the third one is just apply pressure and don't let it off. That's kind of what the Rolling is doing it's putting pressure on and if you have a really bad spike you just hold that spot.

It keeps the weight the pressure on it in the muscle fatigues and eventually has to release it and can't hold it any longer. So that's the classic foam rolling. Then there's roller bars. This is part of the muscle guy. They will have the rollers and all you do is you roll it along the muscle. I love it along the upper calf muscles here the quads. They call them. That feels good. If you want to get the hamstrings you go underneath. Sometimes it's good to do it like this. Sometimes it's good to do it lying down. Getting behind the calf on the sides of the calf is great for doing the legs harder for doing the arms because you don't have your arms to push downward. You have to have somebody do that for you but for things like the forearms I can do pretty good.

If I've been working at the gym I can do it for the biceps. That's actually not bad. If you need a little added pressure just push against something like a wall and use that to kind of hold one side. It's gonna be a while you know as much as you probably get to scrape it, do it out the garage or something like that or on the side of the house. So this type of rolling it's great. When my wife does it she can get my whole back. That's really nice. Great. And then again this is like an eight nine ten dollar Amazon item. I got a kit with a three piece kit. It's got this ball and it's also got the peanut penis two balls stuck together which is good forgetting like the arms or the small the back hitting both sides at once for rolling and then the main roller. That was like a 15 dollar item. So maybe I got twenty five dollars here. Boom.

Here's another great one. This is like a 50 cent item tennis ball. You could roll out an area but you're not going to get a lot of pressure. But sometimes you can just bang it with a tennis ball and that'll release the muscles and break up the fashion a little bit so you can do some tapping. I call it basically pounding on your leg or pounding on an area. You can do that but the classic technique is you take something like a chair. When we get a fresh chair here. Lip locks need a hardship. This is a padded chair. I was going to show you the basic concept of it and all you do is you take the ball and you put it underneath your leg and then just let it sit there and put pressure on it. You can go up and down.

You can let it sit there for a while. That's going to create a release. But the best thing is to be able to roll back and forth maybe over a six inch area three inches forward three inches back and that will grind in almost like the nerve flossing and start to release the fashion then move it forward a little bit to the next spot until you get the entire length of your leg. Perfect. If you can get your leg high enough up that you get a table you can also do the calf as well. So that's a great way to break up those hamstrings just using the tennis ball. Now another great way to do it you would be surprised how much of the tension in your legs in your hamstrings you know part of the reason why you can't touch your toes and have so much flexibility through your legs is actually your feet. So all you need to do is get a tennis ball and not a hard surface.

You could do it in a car but if your carpet's not too thick there's not too much pad on a hard surface, maybe tile floor or linoleum. Simply put the ball down and just start rolling it in. Put it at any spot in your foot. That feels good and then apply some pressure and hold it hold it hold it long as it doesn't hurt you doing it right. You feel some tension there. That's probably where you need it then move it to another spot and just push down on it. Leave it there for a few seconds just as if you're doing a stretch. Do it again in another spot. And what you're going to find is you're going to break up the fashion of the foot. You can release a lot of tendons and tension. A lot of mental tension is stored in your feet if you like acupressure and those types of things reflexology is a lot of those points on your foot.

Some people do this with a spiky ball. They don't do it as hard but the spiky ball will actually stimulate all those acupressure reflexology points. But this is really just to get that release. And if you're a person that's on their feet all day too this can feel fantastic. So you can do it as light or as hard as you want. Again listen to your body, do it very lightly the first time then go a little harder a little higher a little harder see how your feet in your body respond but you may find you have a lot more flexibility from the waist down simply because you use this ball. So that's your bonus tip for today. I'll see you in our very next chapter.

Conclusion

Congratulations on finishing the Book beginner stretching for the inflexible. I made this for people like myself that had difficulty stretching. Now this was originally going to be an hour long training. We obviously went a little bit over that but I always love to give you the extra. So I'm doing this bonus chapter for you to give you still more. I want you to be able to continue learning even after this chaptering is long gone. So keep coming back to it as a resource. But I've got additional resources for you because obviously I couldn't teach you every stretch that's out there or this would be a twenty six week Book. So I'm going to give you some additional resources. Places where you can go to continue your education.

Let's look at some of the first ones now. The first one is beautiful. I love this because they use beach shots and gorgeous scenery. Now this is the pretty girl in the leotard that I told you not to watch but she does a great job of going through all the stretches from a yoga perspective but does virtually every stretch under the sun. Now obviously I want to try to share intelligence. You need to adjust this to your level. But she goes slow. She describes it. She explains it tells you what you should do and what you shouldn't do. So in that way it's perfect training. Check it out I think you're really liking the next one is called rehab my patient. So these are done by physical therapy experts. They're broken down into segments.

A lot of you who are a little bit older like myself or maybe even older than myself into your senior years or maybe even younger and myself. But you've had some difficulties that have caused some of these stretching issues or you just happen to have these difficulties. These are ways that you can go through and learn some physical therapy elements to help deal with different areas. And they also have some stretching chapters as well to continue our theme. I just want to make sure that kind of on every level you're taking care of now guerrilla Zen fitness. This is a little bit of a 50 50 split. I imagine if you're trying to improve yourself, you might want to do a little bit of strength training as well.

So this has stretching and fitness chapters but it also has some weight lifting and strength building chapters perfect for you if that's what you're looking for. Now we've also got yoga with Bird. There are a lot of different people that teach yoga just like butthole fitness. But I think she does a really good job does it nice and slow again is the pretty you're on the leotard but she's a very well trained fitness instructor explains the importance of everything walks you through it does it nice and slow Of course you can always pause the chapters or go back over them but I just think that she does a really nice job and is very comprehensive. So if you have a specific area you want to work on she'll have a chapter for that.

Now some of this is also going to incorporate some fitness type stuff too to not only stretch the muscles but to strengthen them and that should be perfect for you. Now if you're looking to get a little bit more fit and you're my age I'm 55 or maybe younger and me. This is called mad fit. This will take you through and show you all kinds of different great exercises and fitness things that you can do with little or no equipment which is fantastic. So great fitness chapters will give you strength as well as stretching and remember strength supports stretching now if you're my age or a little bit older we've got ones called Senior fitness with Meredith. I like these because she's constantly adding new content.

She takes it slow, she walks you through each exercise she does with minimal equipment, just a few pieces of equipment that you can buy on Amazon or no equipment. So you might have an investment of maybe seventy five dollars if you bought every piece of equipment she shows there certainly no more in one hundred dollars and she respects you. So she understands that if you do senior fitness you might be everywhere from wheelchair bound to fairly athletic for your age. Perfect. So she respects it at all levels and at whatever level you're at you're able to adapt these fitness routines that she's doing to match your level. Now a lot of people ask me how often I should stretch and we really didn't address this in the chapters. So how often does she stretch ? I stretch every single day.

Now why do I do that? Probably about every other day I'm doing a very light stretch which means just enough to a long gait the muscles and alleviate any stiffness that I have. I'm really just gently loosening up the body. You should do that every day so that that fashion doesn't set in place so that your muscles get used to being a long gait but you're not straining them on a daily basis so that's your light day on the heavy day. Maybe every other day or every third day it's up to you. Go ahead and do the heavier stretching where you're trying to make some gains in your stretch a little bit at a time. Remember don't overdo it. One day of overdoing it is going to wipe out at least a week's worth of gains so slow, gentle , easy and steady wins the race.

So one day like one day for games one day like one day for game perfect and Of course stretch and limber up before you do any type of fitness routine. Remember to warm the muscles before you stretch your muscles. Cold muscles tear. Don't forget OK. Those are your bonus tips and bonus resources everybody. Thanks so much. These will show you all my other health fitness resources. I teach in three basic areas. Our old motto was healthy, wealthy and wise.

So I teach psychology and self-help personal development type stuff. I teach business and career development money making type stuff and I also teach the fitness we literally do want to make you healthy, wealthy and wise. If you enjoyed these chapters we have chapters that can help you in virtually every area of your life. That's why I created that motto. Advanced ideas making you healthy, wealthy and what we want. Hit three major areas: your life, health , wealth and wisdom. Thank you so much. You've been fantastic and I'll see you in my very next chapter. Enjoy your bonuses.